I0441107

DIET OF 30 CONSECUTIVE DAYS TO LOWER WEIGHT...With specific advice to maintain a spectacular figure.

Lose up to 15 kilos in just 30 days

Content

Instructions

First step:

1. Eliminate fat and sebum from your face forever

2. Eliminate pimples and acne from your face forever

3. Remove the white and dark spots on your face

4. Shaping your waist

5. Dismantle those walls and accumulated fat in the neck, waist, abdomen and back

6. Clean your skin so that your whole body looks radiant and delicate

7. Disrupt those horrible cellulite or orange peel

8. Remove that dandruff and sebum on the scalp forever

9. Make your hair grow and increase in a surprising way

10. Remove and lift the boot

Annexes:

Instructions

Before starting any diet to lose weight, it is important to know a series of requirements and be clear that success will depend on the discipline and consistency of treatment.

The first step is the detoxification of the organism, so that it can absorb effectively the nutrients of the food that we are going to ingest and that each of the properties of those foods will make its function.

The colon can take days to eliminate waste of previous meals preventing and delaying the passage of the food that is receiving from the small intestine.

The nutrients are absorbed in the small intestine, but if you start a diet with a small intestine full of previous meals the diet will be affected and our effort will be in vain.

It is important to know that you must eliminate desserts and snacks during the period of the diet.

Routine…

First step:

The detoxification

This process will need 3 days, there are many natural supplements in the market that serve to detoxify the organism; You can choose to buy any of them if you prefer, but as it is a completely natural process, here you will have the recipes to prepare your own homemade detox. It should be remembered that there are essential nutrients that can not be missing in your diet and that your body needs it daily to maintain the energy and strength of day to day. During the 3 days it is necessary to drink at least 2 liters of water a day and drink a shake with the following ingredients every morning ½ green apple ½ cucumber A stalk of celery A cup of chopped pineapple.

Blend everything and strain, take this juice in the early hours of the morning.

For breakfast you can choose any of these options: (you can choose two of these)

A boiled egg

One cup of skim milk

A piece of grilled turkey ham

A piece of cream cheese

Optional: a cup of coffee without sugar or low calorie sugar.

At midmorning a cup of fruit, to choose: (pineapple, watermelon, melon, grapes, apple, tangerines, oranges, papaya, strawberries) can mix 3 of these.

At lunch: you should eat an 8-ounce serving of steamed lean meat or steamed fish accompanied by beans and lettuce.

In the afternoon a cup of green tea Every day, both for detoxification and for the routine of the diet ...

15 minutes before dinner put a spoonful of oat flakes in a glass of water and let stand 5 minutes, then take the water carefully not to take the oatmeal seat.

At dinner: you can choose any of the options, just one (liquified strawberries, banana and skim milk, b- liquefied pineapple and cucumber, c- liquefied green apple and orange juice) After the success of detoxification you will start the 30 day routine ...

For the next routine you will have 5 days of diet and at the end of the number 5 you return to number one and repeat the cycle until completing the 30 days.

Diet # 1

Before breakfast

Liquefied green apple with grapefruit juice, strain and take at room temperature or with ice

Breakfast: one cup of whole grain cereal with ½ cup of skim milk

Mid-morning: a slice of watermelon

Lunch: 8 oz. Baked fish, a cup of brown rice and lettuce

Mid-afternoon: ½ green, red or yellow apple.

Dinner: an integral tortilla filled with tomatoes, cucumber, and pieces of steamed chicken breast.

Diet # 2

Before breakfast, cucumber and pineapple smoothie with ½ cup of water

Breakfast: a cup of skimmed yogurt with strawberries

Mid-morning: a cup of green tea

Lunch: a portion of grilled brisket with steamed vainitas and tayotas

Mid afternoon: 2 tangerines

Dinner: a boiled egg, a green boiled banana and a glass of water

Diet # 3

Before breakfast, liquefied pineapple, celery and 3 strawberries with ½ cup of water.

Breakfast: citrus fruits (oranges, tangerines, apples, kiwi, pineapple strawberries, watermelon melon)

Mid-morning: a cup of low-fat yogurt

Lunch: a cup of brown rice with a slice of grilled turkey fillet and tomatoes.

Mid afternoon: a granola cookie and a glass of grapefruit juice

Dinner: 8 ounces of cream cheese with tomato salad.

Diet # 4

Before breakfast, liquefied cucumber and pineapple and a stalk of celery with ½ cup of water

Breakfast: one cup of whole grain cereal with ½ cup of low-fat yogurt

Mid-morning: a banana and 1 glass of water

Lunch: a slice of whole wheat bread with two slices of steamed grouper and salad of beet and lettuce

Mid afternoon: a cup of green tea

Dinner: a boiled egg

Diet # 5

Before breakfast, a glass of grapefruit juice

Breakfast: 8 ounces of cream cheese

Mid-morning: a cup of whole grain and $\frac{1}{2}$ apple.

Lunch: 8 ounces of steamed lean meat with carrots and beans

Mid afternoon: a pineapple and green apple smoothie with $\frac{1}{2}$ cup of water

Dinner: a baked potato with 8 ounces of steamed salmon.

After successfully completing the first 5 days you must return to diet number 1 and repeat the cycle for 30 days.

Important notes: the cucumber must be consumed with everything and its skin, like the potato. You must eat at least 2 liters of water a day and every night 15 minutes before dinner put 2 tablespoons of oatmeal flakes in a glass of water and let stand for 5 minutes, drink the water leaving the oat straw seat in the glass

Diet # 6

Before breakfast. Liquefied green apple with grapefruit juice, strain and take at room temperature or with ice

Breakfast: one cup of whole grain cereal with ½ cup of skim milk

Mid-morning: a slice of watermelon

Lunch: 8 oz. Baked fish, a cup of brown rice and lettuce

Mid-afternoon: ½ green, red or yellow apple

Dinner: an integral tortilla filled with tomatoes, cucumber, and pieces of steamed chicken breast.

Diet # 7

Before breakfast, cucumber and pineapple smoothie with ½ cup of water

Breakfast: a cup of skimmed yogurt with strawberries

Mid-morning: a cup of green tea

Lunch: a portion of grilled brisket with steamed vainitas and tayotas

Mid afternoon: 2 tangerines

Dinner: a boiled egg, a green boiled banana and a glass of water.

Diet # 8

Before breakfast, liquefied pineapple, celery and 3 strawberries with ½ cup of water.

Breakfast: citrus fruits (oranges, tangerines, apples, kiwi, pineapple strawberries, watermelon melon)

Mid-morning: a cup of low-fat yogurt

Lunch: a cup of brown rice with a slice of grilled turkey fillet and tomatoes.

Mid afternoon: a granola cookie and a glass of grapefruit juice

Dinner: 8 ounces of cream cheese with tomato salad

Diet # 9

Before breakfast, liquefied cucumber and pineapple and a stalk of celery with $\frac{1}{2}$ cup of water

Breakfast: one cup of whole grain cereal with ½ cup of low-fat yogurt

Mid-morning: a banana and 1 glass of water

Lunch: a slice of whole wheat bread with two slices of steamed grouper and salad of beet and lettuce

Mid afternoon: a cup of green tea

Dinner: a boiled egg Diet # 10 Before breakfast, a glass of grapefruit juice

Breakfast: 8 ounces of cream cheese

Mid-morning: a cup of whole grain and ½ apple

Lunch: 8 ounces of steamed lean meat with carrots and beans

Mid afternoon: a pineapple and green apple smoothie with ½ cup of water

Dinner: a baked potato with 8 ounces of steamed salmon

Diet # 11

Before breakfast Green apple smoothie with grapefruit juice, strain and take at room temperature or with ice

Breakfast: one cup of whole grain cereal with ½ cup of skim milk

Mid-morning: a slice of watermelon

Lunch: 8 oz. Baked fish, a cup of brown rice and lettuce Mid-afternoon ½ green, red or yellow apple

Dinner: an integral tortilla filled with tomatoes, cucumber, and pieces of steamed chicken breast.

Diet # 12

Before breakfast, cucumber and pineapple smoothie with ½ cup of water

Breakfast: a cup of skimmed yogurt with strawberries

Mid-morning: a cup of green tea

Lunch: a portion of grilled brisket with steamed vainitas and tayotas

Mid afternoon: 2 tangerines

Dinner: a boiled egg, a green boiled banana and a glass of water.

Diet # 13

Before breakfast, liquefied pineapple, celery and 3 strawberries with ½ cup of water.

Breakfast: citrus fruits (oranges, tangerines, apples, kiwi, pineapple strawberries, watermelon melon)

Mid-morning: a cup of low-fat yogurt

Lunch: a cup of brown rice with a slice of grilled turkey fillet and tomatoes.

Mid afternoon: a granola cookie and a glass of grapefruit juice

Dinner: 8 ounces of cream cheese with tomato salad.

Diet # 14

Before breakfast, liquefied cucumber and pineapple and a stalk of celery with ½ cup of water

Breakfast: one cup of whole grain cereal with ½ cup of low-fat yogurt
Mid-morning: a banana and 1 glass of water

Lunch: a slice of whole wheat bread with two slices of steamed grouper and salad of beet and lettuce

Mid afternoon: a cup of green tea

Dinner: a boiled egg.

Diet # 15

Before breakfast, a glass of grapefruit juice

Breakfast: 8 ounces of cream cheese

Mid-morning: a cup of whole grain and $\frac{1}{2}$ apple

Lunch: 8 ounces of steamed lean meat with carrots and beans

Mid afternoon: a pineapple and green apple smoothie with $\frac{1}{2}$ cup of water

Dinner: a baked potato with 8 ounces of steamed salmon.

Diet # 16

Before breakfast Liquefied green apple with grapefruit juice, strain and take at room temperature or with ice

Breakfast: one cup of whole grain cereal with $\frac{1}{2}$ cup of skim milk

Mid-morning: a slice of watermelon

Lunch: 8 oz. Baked fish, a cup of brown rice and lettuce

Mid-afternoon: $\frac{1}{2}$ green, red or yellow apple

Dinner: an integral tortilla filled with tomatoes, cucumber, and pieces of steamed chicken breast.

Diet # 17

Before breakfast, cucumber and pineapple smoothie with $\frac{1}{2}$ cup of water

Breakfast: a cup of skimmed yogurt with strawberries

Mid-morning: a cup of green tea

Lunch: a portion of grilled brisket with steamed vainitas and tayotas

Mid afternoon: 2 tangerines

Dinner: a boiled egg, a green boiled banana and a glass of water.

Diet # 18

Before breakfast, liquefied pineapple, celery and 3 strawberries with ½ cup of water.

Breakfast: citrus fruits (oranges, tangerines, apples, kiwi, pineapple strawberries, watermelon melon)

Mid-morning: a cup of low-fat yogurt

Lunch: a cup of brown rice with a slice of grilled turkey fillet and tomatoes.

Mid afternoon: a granola cookie and a glass of grapefruit juice

Dinner: 8 ounces of cream cheese with tomato salad.

Diet # 19

Before breakfast, liquefied cucumber and pineapple and a stalk of celery with ½ cup of water

Breakfast: one cup of whole grain cereal with ½ cup of low-fat yogurt

Mid-morning: a banana and 1 glass of water

Lunch: a slice of whole wheat bread with two slices of steamed grouper and salad of beet and lettuce

Mid afternoon: a cup of green tea

Dinner: a boiled egg

Diet # 20

Before breakfast, a glass of grapefruit juice

Breakfast: 8 ounces of cream cheese

Mid-morning: a cup of whole grain and $\frac{1}{2}$ apple

Lunch: **8** ounces of steamed lean meat with carrots and beans

Mid afternoon: a pineapple and green apple smoothie with ½ cup of water

Dinner: a baked potato with 8 ounces of steamed salmon.

Diet # 21

Before breakfast. Liquefied green apple with grapefruit juice, strain and take at room temperature or with ice

Breakfast: one cup of whole grain cereal with ½ cup of skim milk

Mid-morning: a slice of watermelon

Lunch: 8 oz. Baked fish, a cup of brown rice and lettuce

Mid-afternoon: $\frac{1}{2}$ green, red or yellow apple

Dinner: an integral tortilla filled with tomatoes, cucumber, and pieces of steamed chicken breast.

Diet # 22

Before breakfast, cucumber and pineapple smoothie with $\frac{1}{2}$ cup of water

Breakfast: a cup of skimmed yogurt with strawberries

Mid-morning: a cup of green tea

Lunch: a portion of grilled brisket with steamed vainitas and tayotas

Mid afternoon: 2 tangerines

Dinner: a boiled egg, a green boiled banana and a glass of water

Diet # 23

Before breakfast, liquefied pineapple, celery and 3 strawberries with ½ cup of water.

Breakfast: citrus fruits (oranges, tangerines, apples, kiwi, pineapple strawberries, watermelon melon)

Mid-morning: a cup of low-fat yogurt

Lunch: a cup of brown rice with a slice of grilled turkey fillet and tomatoes.

Mid afternoon: a granola cookie and a glass of grapefruit juice

Dinner: 8 ounces of cream cheese with tomato salad.

Diet # 24

Before breakfast, liquefied cucumber and pineapple and a stalk of celery with $\frac{1}{2}$ cup of water

Breakfast: one cup of whole grain cereal with $\frac{1}{2}$ cup of low-fat yogurt

Mid-morning: a banana and 1 glass of water

Lunch: a slice of whole wheat bread with two slices of steamed grouper and salad of beet and lettuce

Mid afternoon: a cup of green tea

Dinner: a boiled egg.

Diet # 25

Before breakfast, a glass of grapefruit juice

Breakfast: 8 ounces of cream cheese

Mid-morning: a cup of whole grain and $\frac{1}{2}$ apple

Lunch: 8 ounces of steamed lean meat with carrots and beans

Mid afternoon: a pineapple and green apple smoothie with ½ cup of water

Dinner: a baked potato with 8 ounces of steamed salmon.

Diet # 26

Before breakfast. Liquefied green apple with grapefruit juice, strain and take at room temperature or with ice

Breakfast: one cup of whole grain cereal with ½ cup of skim milk

Mid-morning: a slice of watermelon

Lunch: 8 oz. Baked fish, a cup of brown rice and lettuce

Mid-afternoon: ½ green, red or yellow apple

Dinner: an integral tortilla filled with tomatoes, cucumber, and pieces of steamed chicken breast.

Diet # 27

Before breakfast, cucumber and pineapple smoothie with ½ cup of water

Breakfast: a cup of skimmed yogurt with strawberries

Mid-morning: a cup of green tea

Lunch: a portion of grilled brisket with steamed vainitas and tayotas

Mid afternoon: 2 tangerines

Dinner: a boiled egg, a green boiled banana and a glass of water.

Diet # 28

Before breakfast, liquefied pineapple, celery and 3 strawberries with ½ cup of water.

Breakfast: citrus fruits (oranges, tangerines, apples, kiwi, pineapple strawberries, watermelon melon)

Mid-morning: a cup of low-fat yogurt

Lunch: a cup of brown rice with a slice of grilled turkey fillet and tomatoes.

Mid afternoon: a granola cookie and a glass of grapefruit juice

Dinner: 8 ounces of cream cheese with tomato salad.

Diet # 29

Before breakfast, liquefied cucumber and pineapple and a stalk of celery with ½ cup of water

Breakfast: one cup of whole grain cereal with ½ cup of low-fat yogurt

Mid-morning: a banana and 1 glass of water

Lunch: a slice of whole wheat bread with two slices of steamed grouper and salad of beet and lettuce

Mid afternoon: a cup of green tea

Dinner: a boiled egg.

Diet # 30

Before breakfast, a glass of grapefruit juice Breakfast: 8 ounces of cream cheese

Mid-morning: a cup of whole grain and $\frac{1}{2}$ apple

Lunch: 8 ounces of steamed lean meat with carrots and beans

Mid afternoon: a pineapple and green apple smoothie with ½ cup of water

Dinner: a baked potato with 8 ounces of steamed salmon.

At the end of 30 days you must have lost at least 15 kilos. To maintain the weight achieved return to your previous food routine alternating a normal day and one choosing any of the recipes from 1 to 5. Specific tips to maintain a spectacular figure.

1. Eliminate fat, pimples and acne from your face forever

If you have that face full of grease, sebum and in hot weather seems to be a melted candle. Take a piece of cactus leaf, with care of a few tiny thorn that if they come in contact with your skin they enter and bother you, before using it, scrape it with a knife to remove it. Wash it well, and open it, spread that gel on your face washed with oatmeal soap and dried, leave for 20 minutes and rinse with natural water. Do it 3 times per week. Or more if you think it is necessary, even if your fat is eliminated so much that you will need to hydrate it later.

2. Eliminate blackheads, and acne from your face forever.

Exfoliate 3 times a week with baking soda and water, then put prickly pear.

3. Remove the spots, white a dark of your face

To remove stains from the face Always wash face with soap or oatmeal gel and take a piece of aloe vera, peel and spread gel for 20 minutes three times a week, remove with water and oatmeal soap.

4. **Shape your waist Screw a large towel and lie on the floor in supine position and enter a towel roll at waist level and wait 5 minutes, get up carefully as the bones will ache at the beginning.**

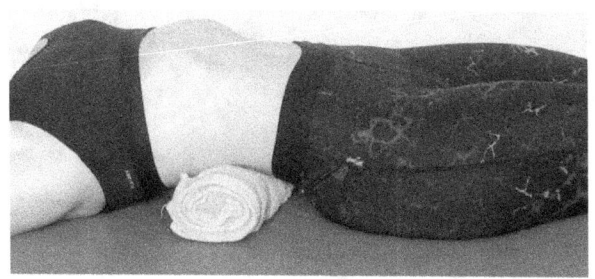

5. Dismantle those walls and accumulated fat in the neck, waist, abdomen and back

a) **Every day.** This must be done before performing the previous exercise. Do crunches down in straight position to touch the fingers of the feet with those of the hands. 60 every day.

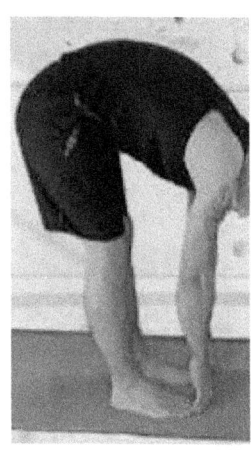

b) **2 cinnamon sticks and 6 grains of malagueta boil daily morning and night.** Take half a green apple when it has boiled, prepare the infusion and remove the cinnamon and maguey, pour into a blender apple and liquid and liquefy, take without straining and without sweetening. It will not be necessary to do it for a long time, in 30 days it will be perfect, even so you can use it longer if you wish.

6. Clean your skin so that everything looks radiant and delicate

Buy a moisturizing bath gel that contains milk and honey, pour a handful of ground coffee and a couple of tablespoons of baking soda and bathe with this every day.

7. Disrupt those horrible cellulite or orange peel

The above recipe will help you eliminate cellulite, yet go to the sauna every 15 days and exfóliate with baking soda, coffee and honey and green oil.

8. Remove that dandruff and sebum on the scalp forever

20 minutes before washing your hair, apply natural gel from the cactus leaf on the scalp. Then wash your hair with shampoo, prepare your shampoo with a little bicarbonate and two tablespoons of apple cider vinegar, use a citrus

condition or indicated for oily hair. Wash your hair twice a week.

9. Make your hair grow and increase in quantity Prepare your dropper:

Gin, a piece of crushed ginger, 2 cinnamon sticks and a juice of guava and rosemary leaves. Let it age 15 days before starting to use it, it is important not to let it fall because it will ferment. Apply it on the skull whenever Wash your hair and do not rinse.

10. Take out your booty Perform 10 sections daily with each leg this exercise of the following image. Support hands on the wall if you want and hold 2 minutes in position changing legs until you complete 5 sections in each one. At first you can do less until you get used to it.

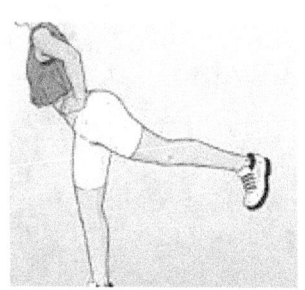

Product images:

Nopal or prickly

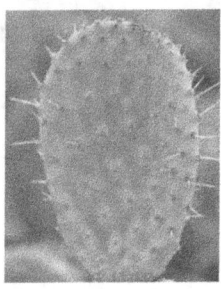

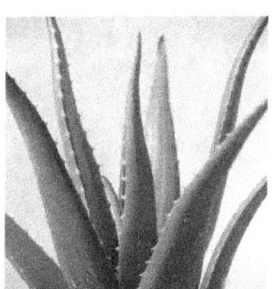

Aloe vera or Aloe

Cinnamon

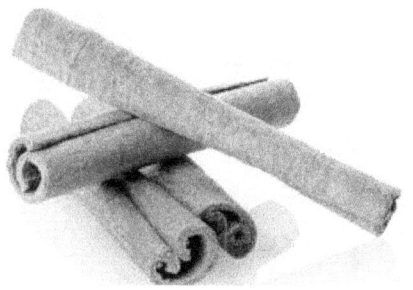

Malagueta

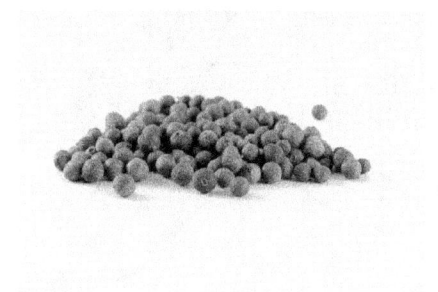

Ginger

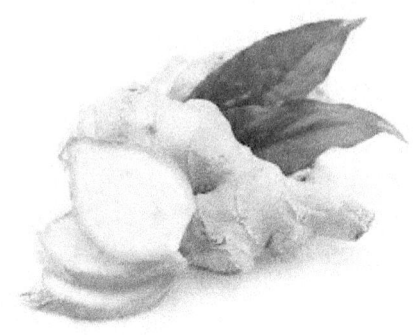

Guava leaves

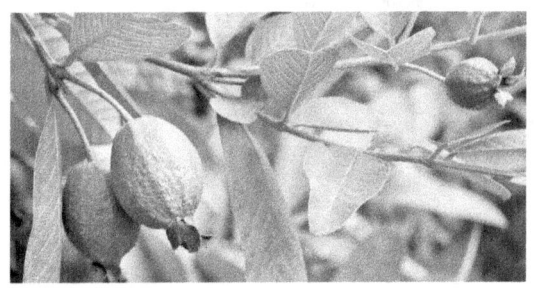

Rosemary

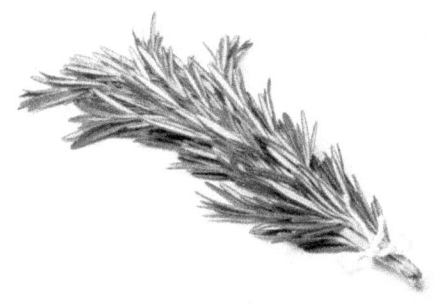

Gin is a type of alcohol similar to white rum

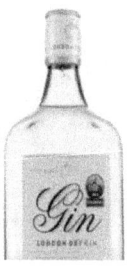

ANNEXES:

Dietary recommendation to maintain the ideal weight

Food Routine:

Having a healthy diet is essential to ensure the normal functioning of our cognitive, physical and online skills. Incorporate healthy habits into your life and you will feel the change

Set schedules for your meals

Ideally, you can set schedules for the four main meals of the day. Mark schedules and respect them will be a great first step to start being healthier.

Chew food slowly

It is not a race, to properly digest the food you must chew for a considerable time. In addition you will feel satiated faster and little by little you will notice how your portions get smaller.

Consume fruits and vegetables

For you to like them, inquire about the way you like them most.

Consume skim or low-fat dairy products.

It is not only about eating well, but about controlling what you eat and choosing the best foods.

Choose products with healthy fats such as olive oil or those that are rich in antioxidants.

Eat fish

It is recommended that you eat fish 3 or more times a week, especially blue.

Take a lot of water

Remember that soft drinks or sodas are very sugary and have a lot of calories.

Practice exercises

Ideally, you can do it four times a week and for about 40 minutes. Remember that there are no miraculous remedies that in a week will make you lose weight.

RECOMMENDED BOOKS IN SPANISH:

De Carmelina Tejada

Disponibles en Amazon:

Serie: Repostería. Cocina y bebidas.

1. 25 ideas para la cena

2. Desayunos y cenas rápidos, fáciles y nutritivos. 60 recetas

3. ¡Desayunos, rápidos, Fáciles y nutritivos para niños y adultos!

4. Curso completo de Repostería. Libro de Repostería

5. Libro completo para Postres. 36 Recetas

6. Panecillos caseros para el desayuno que puedes preparar en casa

Carmelina tejada, R.D.

2019

Derecho de autor registrado

¡Dios te Bendiga!

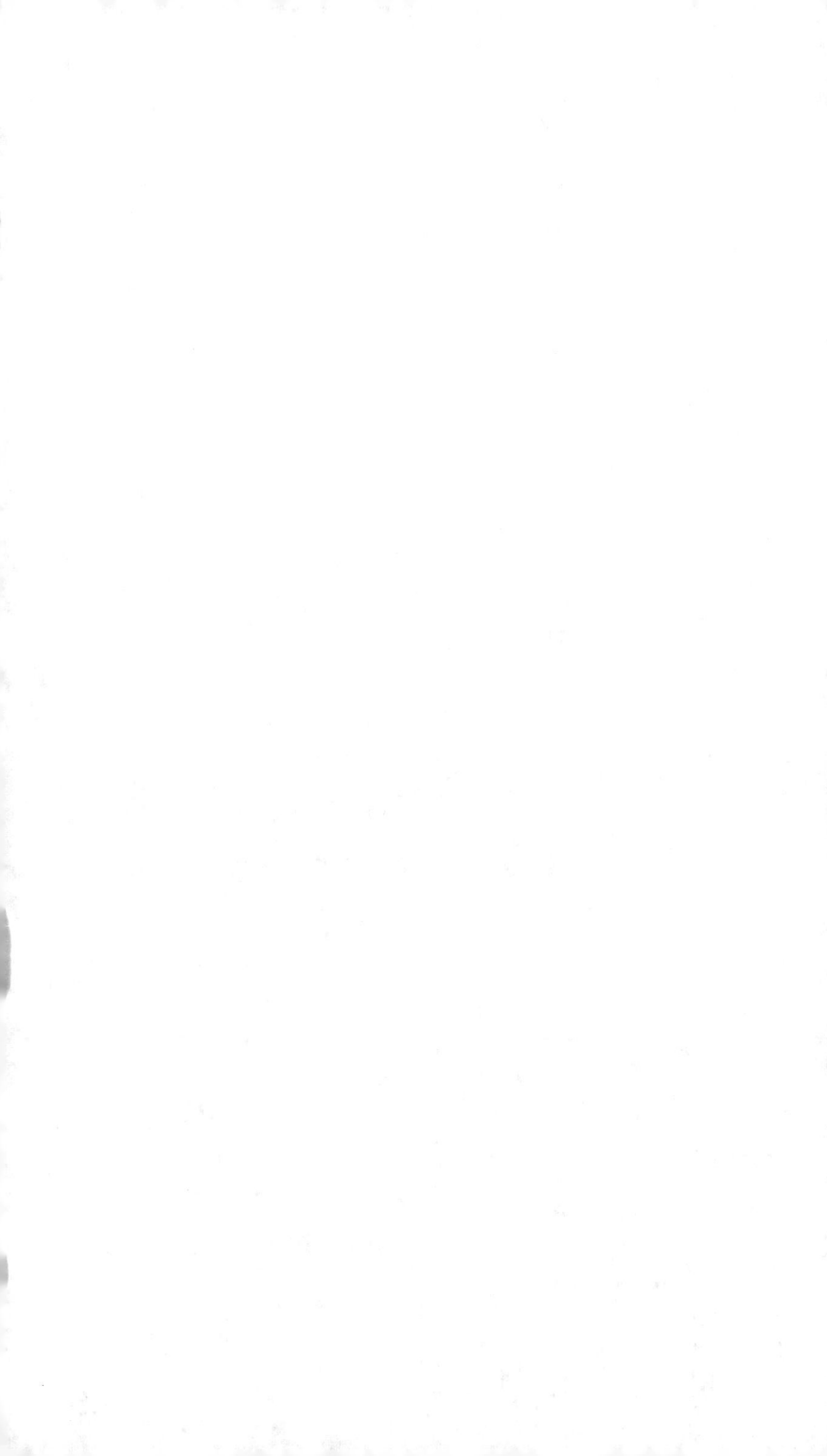

www.ingramcontent.com/pod-product-compliance
Lightning Source LLC
Chambersburg PA
CBHW071241280526
45788CB00004B/1538